Weight Watchers
Diet and Exercise Log

Goals:

30 DAYS: _____

60 DAYS: _____

90 DAYS: _____

Copyright © 2012

All rights reserved.
ISBN: 1495213528
ISBN-13: 928-1495213526

DAY:_____									
WEIGHT:	**POINTS:**		**M**	**T**	**W**	**TH**	**F**	**S**	**SU**

BREAKFAST	**CALORIES**	**POINTS**

LUNCH	**CALORIES**	**POINTS**

DINNER	**CALORIES**	**POINTS**

SNACKS	**CALORIES**	**POINTS**

TOTALS		

STRENGTH TRAINING	**WEIGHT**	**REPS**

CARDIO TRAINING	**TIME**	**DISTANCE**

DAY:_____				
WEIGHT:	**POINTS:**		**M T W TH F S SU**	
BREAKFAST		**CALORIES**	**POINTS**	
LUNCH		**CALORIES**	**POINTS**	
DINNER		**CALORIES**	**POINTS**	
SNACKS		**CALORIES**	**POINTS**	
TOTALS				
STRENGTH TRAINING		**WEIGHT**	**REPS**	
CARDIO TRAINING		**TIME**	**DISTANCE**	

DAY:_____					
WEIGHT:	**POINTS:**		**M T W TH F S SU**		
BREAKFAST		**CALORIES**		**POINTS**	
LUNCH		**CALORIES**		**POINTS**	
DINNER		**CALORIES**		**POINTS**	
SNACKS		**CALORIES**		**POINTS**	
TOTALS					
STRENGTH TRAINING		**WEIGHT**		**REPS**	
CARDIO TRAINING		**TIME**		**DISTANCE**	

DAY:_____

WEIGHT: **POINTS:**   **M   T   W   TH   F   S   SU**

BREAKFAST	CALORIES	POINTS

LUNCH	CALORIES	POINTS

DINNER	CALORIES	POINTS

SNACKS	CALORIES	POINTS

TOTALS		
STRENGTH TRAINING	WEIGHT	REPS

CARDIO TRAINING	TIME	DISTANCE

DAY:_____

WEIGHT: **POINTS:**   **M T W TH F S SU**

BREAKFAST	CALORIES	POINTS

LUNCH	CALORIES	POINTS

DINNER	CALORIES	POINTS

SNACKS	CALORIES	POINTS

TOTALS		

STRENGTH TRAINING	WEIGHT	REPS

CARDIO TRAINING	TIME	DISTANCE

DAY:_____

WEIGHT: _____ POINTS: _____ **M T W TH F S SU**

BREAKFAST	CALORIES	POINTS

LUNCH	CALORIES	POINTS

DINNER	CALORIES	POINTS

SNACKS	CALORIES	POINTS

TOTALS		
STRENGTH TRAINING	WEIGHT	REPS

CARDIO TRAINING	TIME	DISTANCE

DAY:_____					
WEIGHT:	**POINTS:**		**M T W TH F S SU**		

BREAKFAST	**CALORIES**	**POINTS**

LUNCH	**CALORIES**	**POINTS**

DINNER	**CALORIES**	**POINTS**

SNACKS	**CALORIES**	**POINTS**

TOTALS		

STRENGTH TRAINING	**WEIGHT**	**REPS**

CARDIO TRAINING	**TIME**	**DISTANCE**

DAY:_____

WEIGHT:_____**POINTS:**_____**M T W TH F S SU**

BREAKFAST	CALORIES	POINTS

LUNCH	CALORIES	POINTS

DINNER	CALORIES	POINTS

SNACKS	CALORIES	POINTS

TOTALS		

STRENGTH TRAINING	WEIGHT	REPS

CARDIO TRAINING	TIME	DISTANCE

DAY:_____

WEIGHT: _____ **POINTS:** _____   **M T W TH F S SU**

BREAKFAST	CALORIES	POINTS

LUNCH	CALORIES	POINTS

DINNER	CALORIES	POINTS

SNACKS	CALORIES	POINTS

TOTALS		

STRENGTH TRAINING	WEIGHT	REPS

CARDIO TRAINING	TIME	DISTANCE

DAY:_____

WEIGHT: **POINTS:**   **M   T   W   TH   F   S   SU**

BREAKFAST	CALORIES	POINTS

LUNCH	CALORIES	POINTS

DINNER	CALORIES	POINTS

SNACKS	CALORIES	POINTS

TOTALS		
STRENGTH TRAINING	**WEIGHT**	**REPS**

CARDIO TRAINING	TIME	DISTANCE

DAY:_____

WEIGHT: **POINTS:**   **M   T   W   TH   F   S   SU**

BREAKFAST	CALORIES	POINTS

LUNCH	CALORIES	POINTS

DINNER	CALORIES	POINTS

SNACKS	CALORIES	POINTS

TOTALS		
STRENGTH TRAINING	WEIGHT	REPS

CARDIO TRAINING	TIME	DISTANCE

DAY:_____

WEIGHT:_____ POINTS:_____ **M T W TH F S SU**

BREAKFAST	CALORIES	POINTS

LUNCH	CALORIES	POINTS

DINNER	CALORIES	POINTS

SNACKS	CALORIES	POINTS

TOTALS		

STRENGTH TRAINING	WEIGHT	REPS

CARDIO TRAINING	TIME	DISTANCE

DAY:_____				
WEIGHT:	**POINTS:**		**M T W TH F S SU**	
BREAKFAST		**CALORIES**	**POINTS**	
LUNCH		**CALORIES**	**POINTS**	
DINNER		**CALORIES**	**POINTS**	
SNACKS		**CALORIES**	**POINTS**	
TOTALS				
STRENGTH TRAINING		**WEIGHT**	**REPS**	
CARDIO TRAINING		**TIME**	**DISTANCE**	

DAY:_____

WEIGHT:_____ POINTS:_____ **M T W TH F S SU**

BREAKFAST	CALORIES	POINTS

LUNCH	CALORIES	POINTS

DINNER	CALORIES	POINTS

SNACKS	CALORIES	POINTS

TOTALS		

STRENGTH TRAINING	WEIGHT	REPS

CARDIO TRAINING	TIME	DISTANCE

DAY:_____									
WEIGHT:		**POINTS:**	M	T	W	TH	F	S	SU

BREAKFAST	CALORIES	POINTS

LUNCH	CALORIES	POINTS

DINNER	CALORIES	POINTS

SNACKS	CALORIES	POINTS

TOTALS		

STRENGTH TRAINING	WEIGHT	REPS

CARDIO TRAINING	TIME	DISTANCE

DAY:_____

WEIGHT: POINTS: M   T   W   TH   F   S   SU

BREAKFAST	CALORIES	POINTS

LUNCH	CALORIES	POINTS

DINNER	CALORIES	POINTS

SNACKS	CALORIES	POINTS

TOTALS		
STRENGTH TRAINING	WEIGHT	REPS

CARDIO TRAINING	TIME	DISTANCE

DAY:_____

WEIGHT:_____ POINTS:_____ **M T W TH F S SU**

BREAKFAST	CALORIES	POINTS

LUNCH	CALORIES	POINTS

DINNER	CALORIES	POINTS

SNACKS	CALORIES	POINTS

TOTALS		

STRENGTH TRAINING	WEIGHT	REPS

CARDIO TRAINING	TIME	DISTANCE

DAY:_____				
WEIGHT:	**POINTS:**		**M T W TH F S SU**	

BREAKFAST	**CALORIES**	**POINTS**
LUNCH	**CALORIES**	**POINTS**
DINNER	**CALORIES**	**POINTS**
SNACKS	**CALORIES**	**POINTS**
TOTALS		
STRENGTH TRAINING	**WEIGHT**	**REPS**
CARDIO TRAINING	**TIME**	**DISTANCE**

DAY:_____

WEIGHT: **POINTS:**   **M   T   W   TH   F   S   SU**

BREAKFAST	CALORIES	POINTS

LUNCH	CALORIES	POINTS

DINNER	CALORIES	POINTS

SNACKS	CALORIES	POINTS

TOTALS		

STRENGTH TRAINING	WEIGHT	REPS

CARDIO TRAINING	TIME	DISTANCE

DAY: _____

WEIGHT: **POINTS:**   **M   T   W   TH   F   S   SU**

BREAKFAST	CALORIES	POINTS

LUNCH	CALORIES	POINTS

DINNER	CALORIES	POINTS

SNACKS	CALORIES	POINTS

TOTALS		
STRENGTH TRAINING	**WEIGHT**	**REPS**

CARDIO TRAINING	TIME	DISTANCE

DAY:_____					
WEIGHT:	**POINTS:**		**M T W TH F S SU**		
BREAKFAST		**CALORIES**		**POINTS**	
LUNCH		**CALORIES**		**POINTS**	
DINNER		**CALORIES**		**POINTS**	
SNACKS		**CALORIES**		**POINTS**	
TOTALS					
STRENGTH TRAINING		**WEIGHT**		**REPS**	
CARDIO TRAINING		**TIME**		**DISTANCE**	

DAY:_____

WEIGHT:_____ POINTS:_____ M T W TH F S SU

BREAKFAST	CALORIES	POINTS

LUNCH	CALORIES	POINTS

DINNER	CALORIES	POINTS

SNACKS	CALORIES	POINTS

TOTALS		

STRENGTH TRAINING	WEIGHT	REPS

CARDIO TRAINING	TIME	DISTANCE

DAY:_____

WEIGHT:_____ POINTS:_____ M T W TH F S SU

BREAKFAST	CALORIES	POINTS

LUNCH	CALORIES	POINTS

DINNER	CALORIES	POINTS

SNACKS	CALORIES	POINTS

TOTALS		

STRENGTH TRAINING	WEIGHT	REPS

CARDIO TRAINING	TIME	DISTANCE

DAY:_____

WEIGHT:　　　　**POINTS:**　　　　**M　T　W　TH　F　S　SU**

BREAKFAST	CALORIES	POINTS

LUNCH	CALORIES	POINTS

DINNER	CALORIES	POINTS

SNACKS	CALORIES	POINTS

TOTALS		

STRENGTH TRAINING	WEIGHT	REPS

CARDIO TRAINING	TIME	DISTANCE

DAY:							
WEIGHT:	**POINTS:**		**M T W TH F S SU**				

BREAKFAST	CALORIES	POINTS

LUNCH	CALORIES	POINTS

DINNER	CALORIES	POINTS

SNACKS	CALORIES	POINTS

TOTALS		

STRENGTH TRAINING	WEIGHT	REPS

CARDIO TRAINING	TIME	DISTANCE

DAY:_____

WEIGHT: **POINTS:**   **M T W TH F S SU**

BREAKFAST	CALORIES	POINTS

LUNCH	CALORIES	POINTS

DINNER	CALORIES	POINTS

SNACKS	CALORIES	POINTS

TOTALS		
STRENGTH TRAINING	WEIGHT	REPS

CARDIO TRAINING	TIME	DISTANCE

DAY:_____

WEIGHT:_____ POINTS:_____ M T W TH F S SU

BREAKFAST	CALORIES	POINTS

LUNCH	CALORIES	POINTS

DINNER	CALORIES	POINTS

SNACKS	CALORIES	POINTS

TOTALS		

STRENGTH TRAINING	WEIGHT	REPS

CARDIO TRAINING	TIME	DISTANCE

DAY:_____				
WEIGHT:	POINTS:	M T W TH F S SU		
BREAKFAST		**CALORIES**	**POINTS**	
LUNCH		**CALORIES**	**POINTS**	
DINNER		**CALORIES**	**POINTS**	
SNACKS		**CALORIES**	**POINTS**	
TOTALS				
STRENGTH TRAINING		**WEIGHT**	**REPS**	
CARDIO TRAINING		**TIME**	**DISTANCE**	

DAY:_____

WEIGHT: **POINTS:**   **M T W TH F S SU**

BREAKFAST	CALORIES	POINTS

LUNCH	CALORIES	POINTS

DINNER	CALORIES	POINTS

SNACKS	CALORIES	POINTS

TOTALS		

STRENGTH TRAINING	WEIGHT	REPS

CARDIO TRAINING	TIME	DISTANCE

DAY:_____

WEIGHT:_____ POINTS:_____ M T W TH F S SU

BREAKFAST	CALORIES	POINTS

LUNCH	CALORIES	POINTS

DINNER	CALORIES	POINTS

SNACKS	CALORIES	POINTS

TOTALS		

STRENGTH TRAINING	WEIGHT	REPS

CARDIO TRAINING	TIME	DISTANCE

DAY:_____

WEIGHT: **POINTS:**   **M   T   W   TH   F   S   SU**

BREAKFAST	CALORIES	POINTS

LUNCH	CALORIES	POINTS

DINNER	CALORIES	POINTS

SNACKS	CALORIES	POINTS

TOTALS		

STRENGTH TRAINING	WEIGHT	REPS

CARDIO TRAINING	TIME	DISTANCE

DAY:_____									
WEIGHT:	**POINTS:**		**M**	**T**	**W**	**TH**	**F**	**S**	**SU**

BREAKFAST	**CALORIES**	**POINTS**

LUNCH	**CALORIES**	**POINTS**

DINNER	**CALORIES**	**POINTS**

SNACKS	**CALORIES**	**POINTS**

TOTALS		
STRENGTH TRAINING	**WEIGHT**	**REPS**

CARDIO TRAINING	**TIME**	**DISTANCE**

DAY:_____

WEIGHT: POINTS: M   T   W   TH   F   S   SU

BREAKFAST	CALORIES	POINTS

LUNCH	CALORIES	POINTS

DINNER	CALORIES	POINTS

SNACKS	CALORIES	POINTS

TOTALS		

STRENGTH TRAINING	WEIGHT	REPS

CARDIO TRAINING	TIME	DISTANCE

DAY:_____

WEIGHT:_____   POINTS:_____   M T W TH F S SU

BREAKFAST	CALORIES	POINTS

LUNCH	CALORIES	POINTS

DINNER	CALORIES	POINTS

SNACKS	CALORIES	POINTS

TOTALS		

STRENGTH TRAINING	WEIGHT	REPS

CARDIO TRAINING	TIME	DISTANCE

DAY:_____

WEIGHT:_____ POINTS:_____ M T W TH F S SU

BREAKFAST	CALORIES	POINTS

LUNCH	CALORIES	POINTS

DINNER	CALORIES	POINTS

SNACKS	CALORIES	POINTS

TOTALS		

STRENGTH TRAINING	WEIGHT	REPS

CARDIO TRAINING	TIME	DISTANCE

DAY:_____

WEIGHT: **POINTS:**   **M   T   W   TH   F   S   SU**

BREAKFAST	CALORIES	POINTS

LUNCH	CALORIES	POINTS

DINNER	CALORIES	POINTS

SNACKS	CALORIES	POINTS

TOTALS		

STRENGTH TRAINING	WEIGHT	REPS

CARDIO TRAINING	TIME	DISTANCE

DAY:_____				
WEIGHT:	**POINTS:**		**M T W TH F S SU**	
BREAKFAST		**CALORIES**	**POINTS**	
LUNCH		**CALORIES**	**POINTS**	
DINNER		**CALORIES**	**POINTS**	
SNACKS		**CALORIES**	**POINTS**	
TOTALS				
STRENGTH TRAINING		**WEIGHT**	**REPS**	
CARDIO TRAINING		**TIME**	**DISTANCE**	

DAY:_____

WEIGHT: POINTS: M T W TH F S SU

BREAKFAST	CALORIES	POINTS

LUNCH	CALORIES	POINTS

DINNER	CALORIES	POINTS

SNACKS	CALORIES	POINTS

TOTALS		
STRENGTH TRAINING	WEIGHT	REPS

CARDIO TRAINING	TIME	DISTANCE

DAY:_____

WEIGHT:_____ POINTS:_____ M T W TH F S SU

BREAKFAST	CALORIES	POINTS

LUNCH	CALORIES	POINTS

DINNER	CALORIES	POINTS

SNACKS	CALORIES	POINTS

TOTALS		

STRENGTH TRAINING	WEIGHT	REPS

CARDIO TRAINING	TIME	DISTANCE

DAY:_____

WEIGHT: **POINTS:** **M T W TH F S SU**

BREAKFAST	CALORIES	POINTS

LUNCH	CALORIES	POINTS

DINNER	CALORIES	POINTS

SNACKS	CALORIES	POINTS

TOTALS		

STRENGTH TRAINING	WEIGHT	REPS

CARDIO TRAINING	TIME	DISTANCE

DAY:_____

WEIGHT:_____ **POINTS:**_____ **M T W TH F S SU**

BREAKFAST	CALORIES	POINTS

LUNCH	CALORIES	POINTS

DINNER	CALORIES	POINTS

SNACKS	CALORIES	POINTS

TOTALS		

STRENGTH TRAINING	WEIGHT	REPS

CARDIO TRAINING	TIME	DISTANCE

DAY:_____

WEIGHT:_____ POINTS:_____ **M T W TH F S SU**

BREAKFAST	CALORIES	POINTS

LUNCH	CALORIES	POINTS

DINNER	CALORIES	POINTS

SNACKS	CALORIES	POINTS

TOTALS		

STRENGTH TRAINING	WEIGHT	REPS

CARDIO TRAINING	TIME	DISTANCE

DAY:_____			
WEIGHT:	POINTS:	M T W TH F S SU	
BREAKFAST		**CALORIES**	**POINTS**
LUNCH		**CALORIES**	**POINTS**
DINNER		**CALORIES**	**POINTS**
SNACKS		**CALORIES**	**POINTS**
TOTALS			
STRENGTH TRAINING		**WEIGHT**	**REPS**
CARDIO TRAINING		**TIME**	**DISTANCE**

DAY:_____

WEIGHT:_____ POINTS:_____ **M T W TH F S SU**

BREAKFAST	CALORIES	POINTS

LUNCH	CALORIES	POINTS

DINNER	CALORIES	POINTS

SNACKS	CALORIES	POINTS

TOTALS		

STRENGTH TRAINING	WEIGHT	REPS

CARDIO TRAINING	TIME	DISTANCE

DAY:				
WEIGHT:	**POINTS:**		**M T W TH F S SU**	

BREAKFAST	**CALORIES**	**POINTS**

LUNCH	**CALORIES**	**POINTS**

DINNER	**CALORIES**	**POINTS**

SNACKS	**CALORIES**	**POINTS**

TOTALS		

STRENGTH TRAINING	**WEIGHT**	**REPS**

CARDIO TRAINING	**TIME**	**DISTANCE**

DAY:_____

WEIGHT:_____ POINTS:_____ **M T W TH F S SU**

BREAKFAST	CALORIES	POINTS

LUNCH	CALORIES	POINTS

DINNER	CALORIES	POINTS

SNACKS	CALORIES	POINTS

TOTALS		
STRENGTH TRAINING	WEIGHT	REPS

CARDIO TRAINING	TIME	DISTANCE

DAY:_____

WEIGHT: POINTS: M T W TH F S SU

BREAKFAST	CALORIES	POINTS

LUNCH	CALORIES	POINTS

DINNER	CALORIES	POINTS

SNACKS	CALORIES	POINTS

TOTALS		

STRENGTH TRAINING	WEIGHT	REPS

CARDIO TRAINING	TIME	DISTANCE

DAY:_____

WEIGHT: **POINTS:**   **M   T   W   TH   F   S   SU**

BREAKFAST	CALORIES	POINTS

LUNCH	CALORIES	POINTS

DINNER	CALORIES	POINTS

SNACKS	CALORIES	POINTS

TOTALS		
STRENGTH TRAINING	WEIGHT	REPS

CARDIO TRAINING	TIME	DISTANCE

DAY:_____

WEIGHT:_____ POINTS:_____ M T W TH F S SU

BREAKFAST	CALORIES	POINTS

LUNCH	CALORIES	POINTS

DINNER	CALORIES	POINTS

SNACKS	CALORIES	POINTS

TOTALS		

STRENGTH TRAINING	WEIGHT	REPS

CARDIO TRAINING	TIME	DISTANCE

DAY:_____				
WEIGHT:	**POINTS:**		**M T W TH F S SU**	
BREAKFAST		**CALORIES**	**POINTS**	
LUNCH		**CALORIES**	**POINTS**	
DINNER		**CALORIES**	**POINTS**	
SNACKS		**CALORIES**	**POINTS**	
TOTALS				
STRENGTH TRAINING		**WEIGHT**	**REPS**	
CARDIO TRAINING		**TIME**	**DISTANCE**	

DAY:_____

WEIGHT:_____   POINTS:_____   M T W TH F S SU

BREAKFAST	CALORIES	POINTS

LUNCH	CALORIES	POINTS

DINNER	CALORIES	POINTS

SNACKS	CALORIES	POINTS

TOTALS		

STRENGTH TRAINING	WEIGHT	REPS

CARDIO TRAINING	TIME	DISTANCE

DAY:_____

WEIGHT:_____ POINTS:_____   M T W TH F S SU

BREAKFAST	CALORIES	POINTS

LUNCH	CALORIES	POINTS

DINNER	CALORIES	POINTS

SNACKS	CALORIES	POINTS

TOTALS		

STRENGTH TRAINING	WEIGHT	REPS

CARDIO TRAINING	TIME	DISTANCE

DAY:_____

WEIGHT: **POINTS:**   **M   T   W   TH   F   S   SU**

BREAKFAST	CALORIES	POINTS

LUNCH	CALORIES	POINTS

DINNER	CALORIES	POINTS

SNACKS	CALORIES	POINTS

TOTALS		

STRENGTH TRAINING	WEIGHT	REPS

CARDIO TRAINING	TIME	DISTANCE

DAY:_____

WEIGHT: **POINTS:** **M T W TH F S SU**

BREAKFAST	CALORIES	POINTS

LUNCH	CALORIES	POINTS

DINNER	CALORIES	POINTS

SNACKS	CALORIES	POINTS

TOTALS		

STRENGTH TRAINING	WEIGHT	REPS

CARDIO TRAINING	TIME	DISTANCE

DAY:_____

WEIGHT: **POINTS:**   **M   T   W   TH   F   S   SU**

BREAKFAST	CALORIES	POINTS

LUNCH	CALORIES	POINTS

DINNER	CALORIES	POINTS

SNACKS	CALORIES	POINTS

TOTALS		

STRENGTH TRAINING	WEIGHT	REPS

CARDIO TRAINING	TIME	DISTANCE

DAY:_____

WEIGHT: _____ **POINTS:** _____   **M T W TH F S SU**

BREAKFAST	CALORIES	POINTS

LUNCH	CALORIES	POINTS

DINNER	CALORIES	POINTS

SNACKS	CALORIES	POINTS

TOTALS		
STRENGTH TRAINING	WEIGHT	REPS

CARDIO TRAINING	TIME	DISTANCE

DAY:_____

WEIGHT: **POINTS:** **M T W TH F S SU**

BREAKFAST	CALORIES	POINTS

LUNCH	CALORIES	POINTS

DINNER	CALORIES	POINTS

SNACKS	CALORIES	POINTS

TOTALS		

STRENGTH TRAINING	WEIGHT	REPS

CARDIO TRAINING	TIME	DISTANCE

DAY:_____

WEIGHT: POINTS: M T W TH F S SU

BREAKFAST	CALORIES	POINTS

LUNCH	CALORIES	POINTS

DINNER	CALORIES	POINTS

SNACKS	CALORIES	POINTS

TOTALS		

STRENGTH TRAINING	WEIGHT	REPS

CARDIO TRAINING	TIME	DISTANCE

DAY:_____					
WEIGHT:	**POINTS:**		M T W	TH F	S SU
BREAKFAST			**CALORIES**	**POINTS**	
LUNCH			**CALORIES**	**POINTS**	
DINNER			**CALORIES**	**POINTS**	
SNACKS			**CALORIES**	**POINTS**	
TOTALS					
STRENGTH TRAINING			**WEIGHT**	**REPS**	
CARDIO TRAINING			**TIME**	**DISTANCE**	

DAY:_____

WEIGHT: **POINTS:**   **M T W TH F S SU**

BREAKFAST	CALORIES	POINTS

LUNCH	CALORIES	POINTS

DINNER	CALORIES	POINTS

SNACKS	CALORIES	POINTS

TOTALS		
STRENGTH TRAINING	WEIGHT	REPS

CARDIO TRAINING	TIME	DISTANCE

DAY:_____

WEIGHT: **POINTS:**   **M   T   W   TH   F   S   SU**

BREAKFAST	CALORIES	POINTS

LUNCH	CALORIES	POINTS

DINNER	CALORIES	POINTS

SNACKS	CALORIES	POINTS

TOTALS		
STRENGTH TRAINING	WEIGHT	REPS

CARDIO TRAINING	TIME	DISTANCE

DAY:_____

WEIGHT: **POINTS:**   M   T   W   TH   F   S   SU

BREAKFAST	CALORIES	POINTS

LUNCH	CALORIES	POINTS

DINNER	CALORIES	POINTS

SNACKS	CALORIES	POINTS

TOTALS		
STRENGTH TRAINING	WEIGHT	REPS

CARDIO TRAINING	TIME	DISTANCE

DAY:_____			
WEIGHT:	**POINTS:**	**M T W TH F S SU**	
BREAKFAST		**CALORIES**	**POINTS**
LUNCH		**CALORIES**	**POINTS**
DINNER		**CALORIES**	**POINTS**
SNACKS		**CALORIES**	**POINTS**
TOTALS			
STRENGTH TRAINING		**WEIGHT**	**REPS**
CARDIO TRAINING		**TIME**	**DISTANCE**

DAY:_____

WEIGHT: **POINTS:**   **M   T   W   TH   F   S   SU**

BREAKFAST	CALORIES	POINTS

LUNCH	CALORIES	POINTS

DINNER	CALORIES	POINTS

SNACKS	CALORIES	POINTS

TOTALS		

STRENGTH TRAINING	WEIGHT	REPS

CARDIO TRAINING	TIME	DISTANCE

DAY:_____

WEIGHT: _____ POINTS: _____ **M T W TH F S SU**

BREAKFAST	CALORIES	POINTS

LUNCH	CALORIES	POINTS

DINNER	CALORIES	POINTS

SNACKS	CALORIES	POINTS

TOTALS		

STRENGTH TRAINING	WEIGHT	REPS

CARDIO TRAINING	TIME	DISTANCE

DAY:_____

WEIGHT: POINTS: **M   T   W   TH   F   S   SU**

BREAKFAST	CALORIES	POINTS

LUNCH	CALORIES	POINTS

DINNER	CALORIES	POINTS

SNACKS	CALORIES	POINTS

TOTALS		
STRENGTH TRAINING	WEIGHT	REPS

CARDIO TRAINING	TIME	DISTANCE

DAY:				
WEIGHT:	**POINTS:**		**M T W TH F S SU**	

BREAKFAST	**CALORIES**	**POINTS**

LUNCH	**CALORIES**	**POINTS**

DINNER	**CALORIES**	**POINTS**

SNACKS	**CALORIES**	**POINTS**

TOTALS		

STRENGTH TRAINING	**WEIGHT**	**REPS**

CARDIO TRAINING	**TIME**	**DISTANCE**

DAY:_____

WEIGHT: **POINTS:**   **M T W TH F S SU**

BREAKFAST	CALORIES	POINTS

LUNCH	CALORIES	POINTS

DINNER	CALORIES	POINTS

SNACKS	CALORIES	POINTS

TOTALS		

STRENGTH TRAINING	WEIGHT	REPS

CARDIO TRAINING	TIME	DISTANCE

DAY:_____			
WEIGHT:	**POINTS:**	**M T W TH F S SU**	
BREAKFAST		**CALORIES**	**POINTS**
LUNCH		**CALORIES**	**POINTS**
DINNER		**CALORIES**	**POINTS**
SNACKS		**CALORIES**	**POINTS**
TOTALS			
STRENGTH TRAINING		**WEIGHT**	**REPS**
CARDIO TRAINING		**TIME**	**DISTANCE**

DAY:_____

WEIGHT:_____   POINTS:_____   **M   T   W   TH   F   S   SU**

BREAKFAST	CALORIES	POINTS

LUNCH	CALORIES	POINTS

DINNER	CALORIES	POINTS

SNACKS	CALORIES	POINTS

TOTALS		

STRENGTH TRAINING	WEIGHT	REPS

CARDIO TRAINING	TIME	DISTANCE

DAY:_____

WEIGHT: _____ **POINTS:** _____ **M T W TH F S SU**

BREAKFAST	CALORIES	POINTS

LUNCH	CALORIES	POINTS

DINNER	CALORIES	POINTS

SNACKS	CALORIES	POINTS

TOTALS		

STRENGTH TRAINING	WEIGHT	REPS

CARDIO TRAINING	TIME	DISTANCE

DAY:_____

WEIGHT: **POINTS:**   **M   T   W   TH   F   S   SU**

BREAKFAST	CALORIES	POINTS

LUNCH	CALORIES	POINTS

DINNER	CALORIES	POINTS

SNACKS	CALORIES	POINTS

TOTALS		
STRENGTH TRAINING	WEIGHT	REPS

CARDIO TRAINING	TIME	DISTANCE

DAY:_____

WEIGHT: **POINTS:**   **M T W TH F S SU**

BREAKFAST	CALORIES	POINTS

LUNCH	CALORIES	POINTS

DINNER	CALORIES	POINTS

SNACKS	CALORIES	POINTS

TOTALS		

STRENGTH TRAINING	WEIGHT	REPS

CARDIO TRAINING	TIME	DISTANCE

DAY:_____

WEIGHT:_____ POINTS:_____ M T W TH F S SU

BREAKFAST	CALORIES	POINTS

LUNCH	CALORIES	POINTS

DINNER	CALORIES	POINTS

SNACKS	CALORIES	POINTS

TOTALS		

STRENGTH TRAINING	WEIGHT	REPS

CARDIO TRAINING	TIME	DISTANCE

DAY:_____

WEIGHT: **POINTS:**   **M   T   W   TH   F   S   SU**

BREAKFAST	CALORIES	POINTS

LUNCH	CALORIES	POINTS

DINNER	CALORIES	POINTS

SNACKS	CALORIES	POINTS

TOTALS		

STRENGTH TRAINING	WEIGHT	REPS

CARDIO TRAINING	TIME	DISTANCE

DAY:_____

WEIGHT:_____ **POINTS:**_____ **M T W TH F S SU**

BREAKFAST	CALORIES	POINTS

LUNCH	CALORIES	POINTS

DINNER	CALORIES	POINTS

SNACKS	CALORIES	POINTS

TOTALS		

STRENGTH TRAINING	WEIGHT	REPS

CARDIO TRAINING	TIME	DISTANCE

DAY:_____

WEIGHT: _____ **POINTS:** _____ **M T W TH F S SU**

BREAKFAST	CALORIES	POINTS

LUNCH	CALORIES	POINTS

DINNER	CALORIES	POINTS

SNACKS	CALORIES	POINTS

TOTALS		

STRENGTH TRAINING	WEIGHT	REPS

CARDIO TRAINING	TIME	DISTANCE

DAY:_____

WEIGHT: _____ POINTS: _____ **M T W TH F S SU**

BREAKFAST	CALORIES	POINTS

LUNCH	CALORIES	POINTS

DINNER	CALORIES	POINTS

SNACKS	CALORIES	POINTS

TOTALS		
STRENGTH TRAINING	WEIGHT	REPS

CARDIO TRAINING	TIME	DISTANCE

DAY:_____

WEIGHT:_____   POINTS:_____   M T W TH F S SU

BREAKFAST	CALORIES	POINTS

LUNCH	CALORIES	POINTS

DINNER	CALORIES	POINTS

SNACKS	CALORIES	POINTS

TOTALS		

STRENGTH TRAINING	WEIGHT	REPS

CARDIO TRAINING	TIME	DISTANCE

DAY:_____									
WEIGHT:	**POINTS:**		**M**	**T**	**W**	**TH**	**F**	**S**	**SU**

BREAKFAST	CALORIES	POINTS

LUNCH	CALORIES	POINTS

DINNER	CALORIES	POINTS

SNACKS	CALORIES	POINTS

TOTALS		

STRENGTH TRAINING	WEIGHT	REPS

CARDIO TRAINING	TIME	DISTANCE

DAY:_____				
WEIGHT:	**POINTS:**		M T W TH F S SU	

BREAKFAST	**CALORIES**	**POINTS**

LUNCH	**CALORIES**	**POINTS**

DINNER	**CALORIES**	**POINTS**

SNACKS	**CALORIES**	**POINTS**

TOTALS		

STRENGTH TRAINING	**WEIGHT**	**REPS**

CARDIO TRAINING	**TIME**	**DISTANCE**

DAY:_____

WEIGHT:_____ POINTS:_____ M T W TH F S SU

BREAKFAST	CALORIES	POINTS

LUNCH	CALORIES	POINTS

DINNER	CALORIES	POINTS

SNACKS	CALORIES	POINTS

TOTALS		

STRENGTH TRAINING	WEIGHT	REPS

CARDIO TRAINING	TIME	DISTANCE

DAY:_____

WEIGHT:_____ **POINTS:**_____ **M T W TH F S SU**

BREAKFAST	CALORIES	POINTS

LUNCH	CALORIES	POINTS

DINNER	CALORIES	POINTS

SNACKS	CALORIES	POINTS

TOTALS		

STRENGTH TRAINING	WEIGHT	REPS

CARDIO TRAINING	TIME	DISTANCE

DAY:_____

WEIGHT: **POINTS:**   **M T W TH F S SU**

BREAKFAST	CALORIES	POINTS

LUNCH	CALORIES	POINTS

DINNER	CALORIES	POINTS

SNACKS	CALORIES	POINTS

TOTALS		

STRENGTH TRAINING	WEIGHT	REPS

CARDIO TRAINING	TIME	DISTANCE

DAY:_____

WEIGHT:_____ **POINTS:**_____ **M T W TH F S SU**

BREAKFAST	CALORIES	POINTS

LUNCH	CALORIES	POINTS

DINNER	CALORIES	POINTS

SNACKS	CALORIES	POINTS

TOTALS		

STRENGTH TRAINING	WEIGHT	REPS

CARDIO TRAINING	TIME	DISTANCE

DAY:_____

WEIGHT:_____ POINTS:_____ M T W TH F S SU

BREAKFAST	CALORIES	POINTS

LUNCH	CALORIES	POINTS

DINNER	CALORIES	POINTS

SNACKS	CALORIES	POINTS

TOTALS		
STRENGTH TRAINING	WEIGHT	REPS

CARDIO TRAINING	TIME	DISTANCE

DAY:_____

WEIGHT: **POINTS:**   **M T W TH F S SU**

BREAKFAST	CALORIES	POINTS

LUNCH	CALORIES	POINTS

DINNER	CALORIES	POINTS

SNACKS	CALORIES	POINTS

TOTALS		

STRENGTH TRAINING	WEIGHT	REPS

CARDIO TRAINING	TIME	DISTANCE

DAY:_____

WEIGHT: **POINTS:** **M T W TH F S SU**

BREAKFAST	CALORIES	POINTS

LUNCH	CALORIES	POINTS

DINNER	CALORIES	POINTS

SNACKS	CALORIES	POINTS

TOTALS		

STRENGTH TRAINING	WEIGHT	REPS

CARDIO TRAINING	TIME	DISTANCE

DAY:_____

WEIGHT: **POINTS:**   **M   T   W   TH   F   S   SU**

BREAKFAST	CALORIES	POINTS

LUNCH	CALORIES	POINTS

DINNER	CALORIES	POINTS

SNACKS	CALORIES	POINTS

TOTALS		

STRENGTH TRAINING	WEIGHT	REPS

CARDIO TRAINING	TIME	DISTANCE

DAY:_____

WEIGHT: POINTS: **M T W TH F S SU**

BREAKFAST	CALORIES	POINTS

LUNCH	CALORIES	POINTS

DINNER	CALORIES	POINTS

SNACKS	CALORIES	POINTS

TOTALS		
STRENGTH TRAINING	WEIGHT	REPS

CARDIO TRAINING	TIME	DISTANCE

www.ingramcontent.com/pod-product-compliance
Lightning Source LLC
Chambersburg PA
CBHW060434290526
45791CB00002B/948